SANDY WING

STICKING TO A DIET

The Essential Guide For All Things Diet-Related, Discover All the Information About the Different Kind of Diets Available and Learn Which One Would Work Best For You

Descrierea CIP a Bibliotecii Naţionale a României
SANDY WING
   STICKING TO A DIET. The Essential Guide For All Things Diet-Related, Discover All the Information About the Different Kind of Diets Available and Learn Which One Would Work Best For You / Sandy Wing. – Bucharest: Editura My Ebook, 2020
   ISBN

SANDY WING

STICKING TO A DIET

The Essential Guide For All Things Diet-Related, Discover All the Information About the Different Kind of Diets Available and Learn Which One Would Work Best For You

My Ebook Publishing House
Bucharest, 2020

TABLE OF CONTENTS

INTRODUCTION

If you're trying to lose weight and get into better shape, then the first place to look is to your diet. While exercise plays a very important role in our body composition it can't make up for a bad diet. Too many of us think that we can eat unhealthily all day and then use exercise to try and 'make up for it'. That is not how diet works.

This is the first clue that many of us don't really know how diet does work. The next clue comes with the next popular strategy that many people will use to try and get a body closer to the one they always imagined: severely restricting calories or just one food group.

The mistake people make here is that they are thinking of their diet purely as being a source of energy. Your diet is MUCH more than that. Rather than simply being the equivalent of the 'fuel' that a car runs on, it is also the water, the oil and coolant. Moreover, it is also the screws, the nuts, the bolts, the rubber the tires are made of and the glass.

You are what you eat. What you eat is reconstituted and recombined in order to create your body. If you try to lose weight by eating a lot less, then your health will suffer, your energy levels will suffer and ultimately you'll be doomed to failure.

But despite these facts, most of us are still hoping to find some kind of 'quick fix' for our diet. We want some kind of immediate 'cure' for obesity, for lethargy or for spots and we think that the way to get it is simply to change the way we eat.

This is why there are still so many fad diets being promoted on the web. And it is why there are still so many big myths and extreme opinions doing the rounds.

The question is how you can cut through all of this misinformation and all of this bad advice and get to the core of what actually works. That's what we're going to be doing in this book: diet explained.

Because ultimately, losing weight and being in the best shape of your life doesn't have to be complicated and it doesn't have to be hard. It's simply a matter of understanding the science and applying it in a smart way that will work with your routine and that will be easy to stick to.

CHAPTER 1

FOOD GROUPS, CALORIES AND THE DANGERS OF 'A LITTLE KNOWLEDGE'

To understand where all the bad advice and where all the fad diets on the web come from, you first need to understand a little about the history of diet advice and what we have historically thought about our food over the years.

Because this is how things have gone a bit wrong – and it's with the best of intentions.

A long time ago, we didn't know anything about food or about nutrition. We simply knew that eating too much made you fat and eating less made you less fat. Back in those days though we were also much more active and didn't spend most of our time sitting down on the computer.

Over the years though we became more sedentary and at the same time, developed better techniques for studying what food actually did to us. We were thus able to break down our food into major 'groups'.

Those food groups included:

- Carbs
- Fruits and Vegetables
- Fats
- Protein
- Fiber

We learned that each of these food groups would impact the body slightly differently and provide different benefits and weaknesses.

Over time though we would learn that some of these definitions were a little arbitrary (and different versions of this list exist depending on where you look). For example, fruits and vegetables are actually a form of carbohydrate but differ in the way they release sugar into the blood stream owing to their GI index. We'll be looking at that in much more detail in future chapters.

Everything we eat also provides us with micronutrients (amino acids, vitamins, minerals, essential fatty acids etc.) which perform important roles in the body and help build tissues and provide a range of functions. Meanwhile, foods also contain 'calories' which represent the amount of useable energy. The more calories in a particular type of food, the more energy it gives us. If we eat more calories than we burn though, they get converted into fats and stored in the body. To continue the car metaphor a little further, imagine that you were stopping at a gas station but you didn't know when you would next have the opportunity to fuel up. In all likelihood, you would take extra fuel and keep it in a can of some sort as a backup in case you ran out in the middle of nowhere.

Calories were originally worked out as being the amount of energy required to heat one kilogram of water to 1 degree Celsius at sea level. This is still the system we use today. And yes, it is completely arbitrary and outdated at this point.

And if we look at the major food groups, we can see that they each contain a different amount of calories. While carbohydrates and protein both contain 4 kcal (kilocalories) per gram, fats contain 9 kcal per gram.

And seeing as fat is what we're trying to get rid of in the first place anyway, the 'obvious' conclusion to draw from all this would be that we should reduce our intake of fats. Studies meanwhile appeared to show that diets high in fats would lead to heart problems and bad cholesterol and as such, some basic diet guidelines were formed.

The Problem With Modern Advice

Based on this basic knowledge of nutrition, it was established that we should try to:

Limit our overall calories Eat a nutritious diet Avoid fats

This was the advice that most health institutions recommended for a long time – and many still do today. This also includes the NHS in the UK which still recommends low fat diets as being the healthiest way to lose weight.

Meanwhile, this also led to many processed foods being released with fortified mineral and vitamin contents. Eating a vitamin tablet in the morning should be able to provide you with all your required vitamins and minerals and from there you can then eat whatever you want so long as you keep your intake of food low.

As we'll see in a moment, all these conclusions were drawn prematurely and without all the relevant information. Have you ever heard the expression 'a little bit of knowledge is a dangerous thing'? This is the perfect example of that.

CHAPTER 2

THE IMPORTANCE OF FATS, INSULIN AND NUTRITION

While not all of the information we've looked at in the first chapter is wrong, it is wrong to try and form a diet based on that information alone.

This is because it is incomplete and in some cases inaccurate. Let's take a look at calories as a good example.

Because when you think about how they're worked out, you quickly realize that the method is outdated and not particularly helpful. In order for a calorie to mean anything, it needs to be extracted from the food and used by the body. You could argue that a battery can heat a lot of water – but eating batteries won't make you fat… just dead!

Likewise, some foods are easier for the body to use than others and this means that you need to consider more than just the number of calories.

For example, you also need to think about 'GI'. GI stands for 'glycemic index' and it tells you how quickly the energy can be absorbed from your food.

If you eat a simple carb such as a cake or a piece of processed white bread, then this will be digested by the body very quickly. This is man-made, processed food and the body has no trouble breaking it down. While that sounds good though, it actually means that you will then get a sudden and pronounced spike in your blood sugar levels. This in turn means that you'll now have more sugar in your body than you can use in one go and a lot of that will be stored as fat. This can also lower your insulin resistance, eventually causing your body to become less effective at using sugar in the blood.

What's more is that when you spike your blood sugar and then quickly use/store the energy, this causes an equally sudden drop in blood sugar that makes you feel tired and hungry causing you to snack again. And because most processed foods like cake don't contain any nutrients, that means that you'll get cravings for useful nutrients as well.

Decoding the Glycemic Index

Some carbohydrates are more complex and difficult to digest than others and this is where the glycemic index comes in. A value of 100 on the glycemic index is equivalent to pure glucose, while lower levels mean that the food will have a lower and steadier impact on the blood sugar.

If you eat brown, whole-wheat, whole-grain bread then you'll provide your body with a lower GI 'complex carb' and you'll be supplied with a slower and steadier supply of energy throughout the day. You'll be less likely to snack and you won't damage your insulin resistance. What's more is that this food will provide you with more nutrition from the seeds and the germ of the wheat.

The Fall and Rise of Saturated Fat

But you know what else has a low glycemic index? Saturated fat.

The same saturated fat that the NHS still advises you avoid can actually help you to lose weight. Although fat contains more calories than bread for instance, it sits in the stomach longer and releases that energy more slowly. This therefore means you can fill yourself up and stay fuller on a smaller number of calories overall. A little meat or a couple of eggs is much better than a lot of crisps or a lot of chocolate.

What's also important to recognize is that your body won't react to each food group in isolation. If you have a plate of carbs, fats and proteins then they can combine to be digested slower together overall. That means that 'diet food' that removes fat from what you eat is actually a very bad idea.

And this is especially important when you consider that fat has other benefits for the health. Fat is what the body uses to create testosterone (which significantly increases your metabolism and anabolism by the way) and it is what a large proportion of the brain is made from.

But most importantly in this case, saturated fat also aids the absorption of other nutrients. Many key nutrients in our diet are what you call 'fat soluble' meaning that they are absorbed only with the help of fats.

So now consider what actually happens when you eat recommended 'diet food' that is low in fat. Essentially, you are eating the same processed sandwiches but with all the fat removed. That means the total calories will be lower but it means that the sugar content will hit the blood much faster and cause a sudden spike in glucose. This in turn will cause you to feel much tireder much quicker and will cause a lot more of that energy to get stored as fat.

Worse, much of the nutritional value of the food will have been removed and your body will be less able to use a lot of what remains. It's like eating cardboard and it's far less beneficial for you and far less likely to keep you feeling fuller.

And here's the kicker: it turns out that saturated fats probably don't contribute to heart disease or bad cholesterol anyway. More recent studies have used tighter controls to look at the specific effects of saturated fat in the diet and they have largely found that it actually decreases bad cholesterol (low density lipoprotein – LDL) and increases the good kind (high density lipoprotein – HDL).

CHAPTER 3

INTRODUCING THE FAD DIETS, THE GOOD DIETS AND THE ARGUMENTS

This explains to some extent why we have so much contradictory advice available online regarding our diets. You have some people who still promote the 'low fat' advice and you have others that take all this new information to heart and that recommend we completely avoid carbohydrates, or that we avoid simple carbs in particular.

Then there are others that will attempt to use a lot of the information we now have to create 'hacks' that help us to lose weight faster and with less effort.

All of them are wrong and all of them are right. As ever, the answer lies somewhere in the middle.

Let's start by taking a look at some of the most popular approaches to dieting, how they work and what you should take from them…

Low Fat Diets

Low fat diets are diets that haven't gotten the memo about saturated fat. Organizations such as Weight Watchers still recommend this approach and they tell us to eat low fat foods using all manner of scoring systems.

The thing is that you can lose weight on these diets. That's because fat is high in calories and if you're strict enough to ignore the hunger that comes from surviving on a low fat diet, then you can significantly reduce your calories this way so that you are ultimately burning more calories than you are consuming. This makes a deficit and it means that your body is forced to burn fat for energy. Only it's not particularly healthy!

Calorie Counting and IIFYM

A slightly better version of this diet is simply to count calories and to make sure that you consume fewer calories than you burn. This means calculating first the total number of calories you burn in a typical day (called your AMR – more on this later) and then adding up the total number of calories that you are eating. Your aim is then to make sure that you eat fewer calories than you burn off, so that your body will be forced to burn fat stores.

This can and will lose weight loss. As we mentioned earlier, not all of the calories in your food are going to be absorbed and the speed at which they are absorbed can vary greatly. However, if you don't even put enough calories in your mouth to fuel all your activities then you can guarantee that your calorie total will be in a deficit and this means you'll have to burn fat just to stay up and mobile!

Another similar variation on this theme is IIFYM. IIFYM stands for 'If It Fits in Your Macros' and is an approach used by some bodybuilders. This splits calories into the major foodgroups and then defines a set number of calories for each food group. Bodybuilders need 1 gram of protein for every 1 pound of bodyfat in order to maximize their muscle mass. SO if you weigh 175 pounds, that means you need 175 grams of protein or 700 calories' worth of protein.

You can then split your remaining calorie target among the other food groups and aim to complete that.

There are problems with both approaches though. One is that they both force you to calculate and add up all the calories you consume which is a highly time consuming and laborious process – not to mention one that can never be entirely accurate.

Another problem is that it oversimplifies diet and doesn't pay attention to any of the other important factors such as your metabolism, such as your micronutrients or such as the GI of your food. That means that calorie counting can lead to you losing weight in a very unhealthy way. For example, you could lose weight eating nothing but bacon and donuts if it 'fits in your macros'. You'd lose weight yes but you'd also be incredibly unhealthy and probably give yourself diabetes!

The Low Carb/Slow Carb Diet

The other approach that is popular takes an entirely different tact to losing weight and either lowers carb intake, restricts it or completely bans carbs from the diet. This simply demonizes carbs in the same way that we once demonized fats.

By reducing carbohydrates, you can thereby avoid spiking your blood sugar level and maintain a steady level. This in turn means that you will have a steady supply of energy and won't get the cravings or lethargy that comes with sudden spikes and troughs. It also means you can increase your insulin sensitivity and improve your body's ability to use energy in an efficient manner. At the same time, simply by avoiding a lot of carbohydrates like bread, potato, crisps, chips, cake, Coca-Cola etc., you will be able to reduce your intake of 'empty calories' that increase your calories without offering any useful nutrition.

The 'slow carb' diet takes a slightly different approach to this by simply banning 'simple carbs' and focussing instead on complex, low GI carbohydrates such as vegetables and whole grains.

There are problems here though too. For one, the slow carb diet does not guarantee a nutritious meal and nor does it guarantee you'll lose weight. Some people will follow the slow carb diet thinking it's okay to eat as much fat as they like and they'll end up drastically increasing their calories as a result!

Moreover, carbohydrates serve a useful role in the diet just like every other food group does. Low carb diets have been shown to cause low energy and low testosterone and if you're going to be completely strict then avoiding carbs would mean avoiding fruit and vegetables too!

The Paleo Diet

The problem with eating low-fat foods is that they make it harder to absorb the nutrients and don't keep us as full.

The problem with eating simple carbs is that they provide too much sugar and not enough nutrition in return.

And there is one type of fat that definitely does cause heart problems. Trans fat is a man-made fat using hydrogenated oils that causes bad cholesterol and other issues.

Perhaps the problem here isn't the carbs or the fats but rather the fact that they're processed and unnatural.

When we eat natural foods, we are eating foods that our body has evolved to thrive on. As a result, the body is perfectly positioned to be able to absorb all the nutrients. Even the fact that certain vitamins and minerals are included together aids with absorption and makes those foods more potent and more valuable to us. When we eat processed foods though, we don't give our body the sustenance it needs and we can't make full use of the limited nutrition therein.

The paleo diet takes this concept to its natural conclusion by stating that you should only eat foods that would be naturally available in our diet during our evolution. If you could find it by hunting or foraging then you can eat it today.

As a result, you'll end up eating a lot of meats, organ meats, eggs and fish. Lots of nuts, seeds, berries and fruits and lots of vegetables and weeds.

At the same time, you can't eat anything like chocolate, like cake, like bread or like dairy.

This diet works well because it provides the body with lots of nutrition and helps us to avoid processed foods and junk foods. Many people on paleo diets say they feel healthier and more energetic than they have in their entire lives.

But like every one of these fad diets, this one isn't perfect either. These diets make the mistake of sticking too rigidly to the rules. Just because the caveman 'Grok' couldn't eat bread or drink milk doesn't mean that you can't. The evidence conclusively proves that lactose intolerance is only a problem for specific people with a specific allergy not the general public and the same goes for Celiac's disease and gluten sensitivity.

Milk and bread are perfectly fine for you but if you work hard to avoid them, you'll find that your diet becomes very difficult to follow in a modern world and that it's much more likely to fail. Likewise, most people will find it hard to never treat themselves to a chocolate bar. And again, the occasional treat isn't bad as part of a well-balanced diet.

Finally, the paleo diet has the same problem that the low carb diet has – a lack of control means you can still damage your weight if you're eating too much. Contrary to popular belief it's possible to be healthy and overweight!

Intermittent Fasting

Intermittent fasting takes a slightly more extreme approach to the bloodsugar issue in an attempt to accomplish essentially the same thing while at the same time lowering the total caloric intake.

The idea of intermittent fasting is to fast for short periods and to alternate between this and periods of eating normally. This might mean that you stop eating after 4 pm, or it might mean that you attempt the '5:2 diet' and fast for two days of the week consuming only 500-600 calories on those days.

The idea behind this is partly to force a lower calorie intake for the week. At the same time though, it also forces you to lower your blood sugar significantly during those periods, increasing your insulin sensitivity, the function of your mitochondria and your ability to burn through fats. You'll also reduce your glycogen stores and triglycerides by burning through energy when your blood sugar is that low.

The biggest problem with this diet is how impractical it is to stick to. It's also a rather extreme measure which could potentially upset the hormone balance for those who have existing problems.

Mediterranean Diet

Remember when fat was the enemy and everyone thought it caused heart problems?

One of the studies that managed to topple this notion was a survey that looked at the health of people who ate different diets in different countries. It was found here that despite eating a high fat diet, people who lived on the Mediterranean (Italians, French, Greek) all lived longer and had better heart health than those in the UK and US.

Why?

We now know that this is partly because fats aren't that bad for us. What we also know is that the Mediterranean diet is very high in fresh fruits and vegetables, as well as fish, meats, salads and nuts. Those on the Mediterranean actually make food an important part of their day and take the effort to cook fresh, delicious meals to enjoy with their families. These include tons of cancer and age-fighting antioxidants that absorb all the better thanks to the fat and oil content. Because you're filling up on good food, you'll also be less likely to feel hungry and need to snack later on.

This is a great diet to try out but again the problem is that there's very little structure to it, making it all too easy to end up accidentally getting fat on all that healthy food.

CHAPTER 4

THE MIDDLE WAY – HOW TO TAKE
A BALANCED APPROACH TO YOUR DIET

I've explained all of this so that you have a proper understanding of your diet and of the various different views and stances out there. This will help you to better appreciate the benefits of taking a 'middle way' approach that borrows the best elements from each diet without being too extreme or dogmatic.

So here's what we know and what we can take away from everything we've learned so far:

You will lose weight if you burn more calories than you consume All food groups play important roles in the body

A diet is only useful if you are able to actually stick to it It's very important to fuel yourself with lots of nutrients 'Real' food helps you to feel fuller for longer

Processed foods tend to be high GI and offer less nutrition

Spiking your blood sugar damages your insulin sensitivity and makes you hungrier

So taking all this into account, how should we approach our diet?

The first thing to do is to 'roughly' count calories. Creating a calorie deficit is still the best way to reduce your weight and to burn body fat so if that's your aim, then it's a good idea. As you'll see though, there's no need to laboriously count out every single calories – especially seeing as the number is a rough guide to start with!

To do this then, you're going to work out your AMR or your 'Active Metabolic Rate'. This is the amount of calories you burn in a typical day, taking into account how active (or inactive) you are as well as your bodyweight and various other factors.

To work this out, you first start with your BMR. Your BMR is your 'Basal Metabolic Rate' which tells you just how many calories you would burn if you simply sat down all day. Our body needs to carry out a large number of processes simply to stay alive and these include things like blinking, breathing, beating our heart and repairing tissues.

Your active metabolic rate then simply tells you how much you're burning on top of this number by moving. Even if you don't actively work out, chances are that you walk around, go shopping and engage in other basic activities that will increase the amount of calories you burn. This gives your AMR and that in turn should roughly tell you how many calories you use up every day.

To calculate this number, use the following formulas: Men:

BMR = 66 + (6.23 x weight in pounds) + (12.7 x height in inches) – (6.8 x age in years)

Women:

BMR = 655 + (4.35 x weight in pounds) + (4.7 x height in inches) – (4.7 x age in years)

To turn this into your AMR, you then multiply that amount by:

- 1.2 if you're sedentary (little or no exercise)
- 1.375 if you're lightly active (you exercise 1-3 times a week)
- 1.55 if you're moderately active (you exercise or work about average)
- 1.725 if you're very active (you train hard for 6-7 days a week)

- 1.9 if you're highly active (you're a physical laborer or a professional athlete)

Now you have your AMR, your objective is to limit your caloric intake to be lower than this amount. This is where many people would start counting calories, which in turn is what drives many people mad and causes them to fail in their ambition to lose weight!

So instead, aim to calculate only a very rough estimate of how many calories you consume and look at the calories included in all the things you eat regularly. Most of us will circulate between 10-20 meals that we enjoy cooking and will eat a relatively consistently lunch and breakfast.

Now find what the biggest contributors to your overall calorie intake is. Maybe there's a pizza you often eat that is adding an insane 1,500 kcal to your total. Maybe you're drinking a lot of Coca-Cola! Identify these and eradicate them from your diet.

Another tip that you can use is to give yourself a set breakfast and lunch. This works because it will allow you to know exactly how many calories you will have consumed by dinner. If you keep this number low, then you can make sure that you have lots of 'leeway' to be a bit careless for dinner.

For example, if you know that your target calorie intake is 2,000 then you can choose a set breakfast and lunch that will give you a combined total of 700 calories. This then means you have 1,300 calories to consume for dinner before you'll risk gaining weight. You'll pick meals that aren't obscenely high in calories and that will allow you to eat without needing to actually calculate anything at all.

And why are we choosing breakfast and lunch to be the 'static' meals? Simple: because breakfast and lunch are not social meals. When it comes to diet 'adherence' one of the biggest challenges is always the social aspect of eating. It's hard to eat a healthy, boring meal if you're out with friends or on a date. So eat boring when you're in a rush and then sit down to really enjoy your dinners with your family just like they do on the Mediterranean!

Choosing the Right Food

Using this method, you can now maintain a calorie deficit relatively consistently without having to do too much counting, tracking or stressing.

What's important at the same time though is to think carefully about the types of foods you're consuming and how this is going to contribute to your hunger/satiety as well as your overall health.

The aim here is to aim for quality, natural foods that you enjoy but to eat less of them – rather than trying to eat the usual amount of food but getting it from 'low fat' sources.

Try to avoid simple carbs unless you're getting a lot in return (smoothies being one good exception) and look out for nutrient dense 'super foods' like seaweeds, berries and other things that pack a lot of nutrients into a small amount of food. This is what's going to enable you to stick to your goals and it's what will ensure your metabolism works well and your health is at its optimum.

So instead of eating Coco Pops for breakfast, try eating oats. This will release energy slower throughout the day and offer more nutrition. Drink full fat milk so that you absorb the nutrients efficiently and so that you get all the health benefits that come from it.

Likewise, avoid junk sandwiches for lunch and instead look for a salad bar where you can have some salad leaves, fruits and vegetables, nuts and eggs. Swap your morning coffee with cream for a healthy vegetable smoothie.

When you eat dinner, always aim to cook your meals fresh if you can. Think of this like a computer game where the micronutrients you can get in your diet are 'power ups' that will make you stronger, faster, smarter and thinner.

By doing this, you'll be fuelling your body with everything it needs to be healthy, energy efficient and immune to many diseases. You'll also be avoiding spiking your blood sugar too much and this will keep your insulin sensitivity high too.

Sometimes you'll want to have an unhealthy, processed snack and that is fine. As long as you eat lots of other low GI food at the same time to slow the absorption and as long as you're staying under your calorie target and getting all your nutrition from elsewhere – no one is perfect! Meanwhile, don't bother avoiding milk or bread. If you must create a single 'rule' for your natural food, then expand the definition of 'natural' to include anything that could be farmed.

You see it's not really that hard. In many ways you're doing exactly what they did back in the early days of our understanding of diet: eating the same diet but in lower quantities. The difference is that we know why it works and we have a little more control over how we do it.

Science has gone full circle from telling us to hack our diet all the way to telling us to eat as naturally as possible and to sit down and enjoy your food!

CHAPTER 5

THE ROLE OF EXERCISE – INTRODUCING HIIT AND RESISTANCE TRAINING

We said earlier that you couldn't use exercise as a way to make up for a bad diet. While this is certainly true though, that doesn't mean that you can't combine exercise with the right diet in order to maximize your results. In fact, this is something that is very much advisable!

The most obvious reason that you should incorporate some kind of training into your routine along with your new diet, is that it will help you to burn more calories and to significantly increase your AMR. It's often said that the majority of the calories you burn in a day are not burned during exercise.

This is certainly true but it does not mean that you can't also burn an awful lot of additional calories by exercising in the right way.

In fact, if you exercise correctly, then you can expect to burn anything from 400 up to 700 or even 1,000 calories. Seeing as the average AMR is around 2,000 calories this is enough to make a huge difference – allowing you to consume an additional 50% on top of what you're currently eating!

The best way to do this is by jogging and if you incorporate running for 5-6 miles a couple of times a week, then you can actually change your AMR significantly.

This also means that you can get more nutrients and more crucial materials into your body without exceeding your calorie target.

What we're also going to see is that you can smartly use exercise in order to trigger some changes in the body and that this will help you to accelerate your body recomposition even more effectively.

Introducing HIIT

We said we were going to be taking the best elements from all the popular diets and combining them into one superior strategy. So where is the intermittent fasting?

Well actually, we're going to accomplish something similar and lower our blood sugar through our exercise instead.

Traditionally, cardiovascular exercise was once used in a 'steady state' manner. This meant you would run on a treadmill or down the road and you would keep moving for 20, 30 or 40 minutes until you gave up at a steady speed. To accomplish this, you would maintain a heartrate of around 70% MHR (max heart rate). In other words, you wouldn't go 'all out'.

The idea for this was a) that it would allow you to train for longer without collapsing and b) that it would let you burn more fat. Because the body has three different energy systems and it's the 'aerobic system' that we use to burn fat. The aerobic system kicks into play only when we exercise for an extended duration of time and it allows our body to circulate oxygen around the body to break down stored fat tissue and bring it to the muscles. This is why you start panting after a few minutes of light exercise.

But this process takes time and if you are sprinting, then you will need to get energy into your body before you the aerobic system can get it there. This means that you'll then be relying on glycogen stores as well as ATP in the muscle for energy – and not burning fat. This is called 'anaerobic exercise' – i.e. 'not aerobic'.

But HIIT turns this idea on its head and combines both aerobic and anaerobic exercise into one effective routine. It does
36

this by challenging you to train for brief stints (a minute or two) at 90-100% MHR and then to recover for a few minutes by training at a slower pace. So you can sprint for 1 minute, then jog lightly for 3 minutes and then sprint for a subsequent minute and repeat.

This then means that you'll be using up all of the glycogen stores, all of the ATP and all of the blood sugar available to you during the anaerobic portion of your exercise and this will then force you to burn even more fat even more effectively during the aerobic portions of your training.

What's more is that you can trigger something called an 'after burn' effect. This means that you'll have zero energy left that's immediately available after training and you'll thus be forced to burn fat throughout the day. This means that HIIT training can actually help you to raise your metabolism throughout the day and burn more fat.

Resistance Training

If you really want to burn fat though, you should try lifting weights. This is something that many people keen to get thinner won't consider but in fact it is one of the best ways to lose weight and to get thin.

The reason is firstly because weight training itself is surprisingly cardio intensive. By lifting weights you are burning calories and forcing yourself to work hard. The fact you have to push against resistance means you need to recruit more muscle fiber which uses more energy. This is then even more effective if you combine HIIT with resistance training so that you are calling upon your muscle fiber rapidly and for an extended period. This is called 'resistance cardio' and a perfect example is the kettlebell swing. Try using the kettlebell swing with a tabata protocol and you will burn a lot of calories and build a lot of muscle.

But the other thing about resistance training is that it can trigger a hormonal response. When you exercise using resistance training, you'll break down muscle and you'll cause a build up of blood and metabolites in the muscle. Metabolites include the likes of growth hormone and testosterone - chemicals that instruct the body to grow and repair tissue.

When this happens and you then supply the body with an ample supply of protein, it causes you to build more muscle. What's more though, is that this process causes more calories to be sent to the muscle to fuel glycogen stores rather than to be stored as fat. Further, the process of building and maintaining muscle will cause you to burn more calories even when you're resting – it will significantly increase your BMR.

Apart from anything else, the type of body that most people dream of is more the result of toning muscle than it is of burning fat and getting thin. Focus on body recomposition and not weight loss per say!

CHAPTER 6

WHY AREN'T I LOSING WEIGHT? INDIVIDUAL DIFFERENCES AND GETTING STARTED

Now comes the nasty surprise: you can follow all of this advice and do everything we've discussed right down to the letter. But that doesn't necessarily mean that you're going to lose the weight. Or what you might find is that someone else performing the exact same exercise routine and eating the exact same diet is able to lose more weight than you. So what is going on?

This can come down to several factors but it essentially boils down the simple fact that everyone is different. And what works for one person will not necessarily work for another.

One reason for this is the fact that we are all genetically and hormonally different. Consider the huge impact that testosterone and thyroid hormones could have. You might think that hormones are just an 'excuse' for people who can't control their eating but then consider how hard it is for someone with polycystic ovaries or hypothyroidism to lose weight and how tired they feel.

Likewise, think about how lean and ripped someone who uses testosterone can become. This is why some people are naturally mesomorphs, some are endomorphs and some are ectomorphs.

You might not fall into either of those categories but we all have completely unique hormone profiles and this isn't reflected when you calculate your BMR. You might have an actual condition or you might have a borderline condition.

So what do you do? The best options are to restrict your diet even further and try even harder and to look at things you can do to change your hormones and your metabolism. If you have low testosterone for example, there are many diet changes and lifestyle changes you can use to change this. If you have a slow metabolism, look at ways to ramp this up by increasing your insulin sensitivity. Perhaps IF is right for you? With a little advice from your doctor of course.

This is once again why it's so important to consider more than just calories in your diet. A good diet should make you more and more efficient at burning fat. But consider as well that some elements are going to be somewhat genetically predetermined. It's better to try and play the hand you're dealt than it is to fight your genetics and be constantly exhausted as a result.

Routine

There's another aspect that can vary from one person to another and have a big impact on weight loss too and that's routine. Earlier we rubbished the idea that exercise didn't make an impact at all compared with lifestyle.

While that's not the case it is still true that the majority of calories you burn will be burned during other activities.

So if you're doing the same workout routine and being strict with your diet but you don't lose weight as quickly as everyone else, what might be the problem? It may just be that other people are burning calories on their walk to work, or even at work if they do a physical job. If you spend 8 hours a day sitting and you aren't that active the rest of the time… well then you won't lose weight as quickly as someone who works on a construction site or who walks to work 20 minutes there and back every day. This is where using a fitness tracker or something similar to track your actual calories burned at each point can make a big difference.

So with all this in mind, it's important to tweak your diet and routine to work around your routine and around your genetics. Start with this basic diet but use what you've learned to identify what's working and what isn't. With some iteration and measurement you can eventually hope to land on a solution that works for you.

Printed by Libri Plureos GmbH in Hamburg,
Germany